Ultimate Alkaline Foods Guide!

Alkaline Foods

Learn How To Alkalize Your Body With This PH Balance Diet And Superfoods Guide To Increase Your Energy, Fat Loss, Natural Beauty And Health!

Sarah Brooks

STOP!!! Before you read any further....Would you like to know the Secrets of Body Transformation?

If your answer is yes, then you are not alone. Thousands of people are looking for the secret to rapidly burn body fat, keep the weight off, become healthier, and truly transform their body and life for good.

If you have been searching for these answers without much luck, you are in the right place!

Not only will you gain incredible insight in this book, but because I want to make sure to give you as much value as possible, right now for a limited time you can get full **100% FREE access to a VIP bonus EBook** entitled **THE 7 KEYS TO BODY TRANSFORMATION!**

Just Go Here For Free Instant Access:

www.liveFitVIP.com

Legal Notice

Disclaimer Notice

Table Of Contents

Introduction

I want to thank you and congratulate you for purchasing the book, *Alkaline Foods: Ultimate Alkaline Foods Guide! Learn How To Alkalize Your Body With This PH Balance Diet And Superfoods Guide To Increase Your Energy, Fat Loss, Natural Beauty And Health!*

This book contains proven steps and strategies on how you can change your diet to something healthier and better for you in the long-term. With the alkaline diet, your body will function better. The diet plan can also help raise your energy level and improve your immunity to different illnesses as well as infections.

You may not notice it but the foods that you consume on a daily basis have a direct effect on your body, starting with how energetic you are to how your skin looks. The thing is that the average Western diet is actually highly acidic and this causes a number of different health problems for people with heart diseases and obesity being the most common. However, with a simple diet change you can avoid these completely.

We hope that this book can provide you with all the information that you need when it comes to getting started with the alkaline diet and use it to enjoy a healthier and more satisfying life.

Thanks again for purchasing this book, I hope you enjoy it!

Chapter 1: What Are Acidic Foods And How Do They Affect Your Body?

When it comes to maintaining your overall health and well-being, the foods that you consume regularly play a significant role. Too much of acidic foods can bring about a number of health issues just as too much alkalinity can bring about an imbalance. Making sure that your body's blood pH stays within the right level is imperative if you want to stay healthy and avoid different health complications. To do that, however, you will need an understanding of what alkaline and acidic foods are along with the effects they have on your body.

What are Acidic Foods and How Do they Affect your Body?

Contrary to what most people think, simply eating acidic foods will not immediately cause your blood, stomach or body to become acidic too. It is the process of digestion that eventually takes it up a notch and causes damage on your body slowly but surely. During digestion, the stomach secretes hydrochloric acid (a highly acidic substance) and this, mixed with the acid in the foods you eat, will make you feel ill.

Here's a quick summary of some of the most common problems that are associated to having a highly acidic diet:

- If left untreated, high amounts of acid in your body will also begin to move into your tissues and joints. This will not only cause damage but some discomfort as well. In more advanced cases, joint pain is not an unusual symptom. Your bones will also start to weaken more and you will become more prone to bone-related issues such as osteopenia.

- Acidity can also bring about number of skin-related issues; eczema is the most common skin disorder of all. Too much acidity can also lead to brittle hair, dry skin, as well as a number of oral issues. Bleeding gums and bad breath are also common symptoms of a highly acidic diet.

- There are also certain heart issues that may arise from having a highly acidic diet. Two of the most common symptoms would be an increase in your heart rate and arrhythmia. Of course, a highly acidic diet that is coupled with a lack of proper exercise can certainly lead to even greater issues.

- When it comes to the negative effects of too much acidity to your body, your intestinal and gastric systems will take the hardest hit. In some cases, vomiting, nausea, diarrhoea, heartburn and acid reflux may be experienced. This is especially so if there's a major imbalance in your blood PH. None of these are a walk in the park and they usually happen out of the blue as well.

Chapter 2: What Are Alkaline Foods And How Do They Affect Your Body?

We've already made it clear that it is hard to tell which foods are acidic at first glance, even at first taste. The same idea applies to alkaline foods because everything changes once you consume it and once your body begins breaking it down. For example, you'd think that lemons are highly acidic considering their sour flavour, right? Yes, they do contain citric acid but that only matters a little once the food passes through your kidneys.

In this case, lemons are actually quite alkaline. In fact, they are often used for making alkaline water-- a great alternative when you are trying to wean yourself off of flavoured and carbonated drinks.

So now, let's talk about benefits. Your body needs to achieve the proper pH balance in order for everything to function properly. Through the right diet, this can be easily achieved and some of the changes you'll see include the following:

1. Better energy levels – We've already talked about how being acidic can bring your energy levels down, making you lethargic and quite unproductive. If you can get your diet to be more alkaline, however, the opposite happens. Because your cells are healthier and more capable of transferring oxygen throughout your body, you also get a lot more energy. Basically, having healthy cells translates to a fitter and more efficient you. So if you're looking for an energy boost, grab some veggies or an alkaline smoothie instead of another chocolate bar.

2. Improved Immunity – Now, healthy cells also mean that they are more effective in absorbing the nutrients that your body needs from the foods you eat. They are also better in getting rid of any waste products as well as in eliminating any organisms that may make you ill. Of course, if they're not healthy, all of those things begin to deteriorate, thus leaving you more vulnerable to different infections, illnesses and so on. If you're more prone to getting sick these days, it could be that you need to tone down your consumption of acidic foods before things get worse.

3. Youthful skin and glow – When your cells are not constantly being subjected to an acidic environment, they function better and more efficiently. This can also slow down aging. Are you aware that an acidic diet can cause your hair to fall out, your nails to become brittle, your skin to become flaky and make you more prone to acne breakouts? Well, you can eliminate those issues with just a simple diet change. An alkaline diet will also help detoxify your body, thus effectively ridding you of anything harmful and give your skin a more youthful glow.

4. Stronger bones – As you age, your bones tend to become less flexible and more brittle. This is why many people take calcium supplements to help prevent this from happening or at the very least, slow the process down. However, you can prematurely develop different bone issues that will only worsen as you age further. An acidic diet is detrimental to your bone health as it actually eats away the calcium stored in your bones. So despite your best efforts to replenish it by taking the supplements, you will still end up with very little if you don't switch to a healthier diet.

5. Better circulation – Eating alkaline foods and properly balancing your blood pH levels can also help in improving your circulation which then leads to a number of different benefits. Among them are better heart health and a lower risk of developing different heart-related issues. Couple this with a regular exercise routine and you'll also be able to lower the risks of strokes, heart attacks and so on.

Chapter 3: Understanding The PH Balance Of Your Body And The Ideal Levels Of Alkaline/Acid Balance

What does pH mean? PH is basically an abbreviation for "potential hydrogen". As it applies to your body, the higher the pH is, the more oxygen rich the blood is. It is also more alkaline. However, the lower it is, the more acidic and oxygen deprived the blood is. This is when problems begin to arise.

So what is the right balance between alkalinity and acidity?

1. The ideal blood pH would be around 7.4 which makes it just a bit more alkaline.

What happens if the number increases or decreases?

2. Well, it must be noted that even the slightest change can be quite devastating to the body. For example, should it move to 6.8 or 7.8, your cells will soon begin to cease to function and this may result to death.

As always, balance between the two is important and as such, a diet that promotes this balance is necessary for your overall well-being.

**Note that on the pH scale, each number would represent a difference of tenfold each time you go up or down. For example, a pH of 4 would be ten times more acidic when compared to a liquid with a pH of 5.

Chapter 4: What Percentage Of Your Diet Should Be Alkaline Foods?

As you can see, becoming too alkaline can be dangerous as well and as such, it is important to make sure that you don't go beyond the recommended percentage.

<u>So what should the ratio be when it comes to acidic and alkaline foods?</u>

- Experts believe that the ideal ratio for this would be 80% alkaline and 20% acid.

<u>What does that mean for your body?</u>

- This should provide you with just the right amount to balance your blood pH and at the same time, not deprive you of the vitamins, minerals and nutrients that you need on a daily basis. This is also the thing that makes it one of the better weight loss diets out there.

  Since it's all about balance, you need not restrict yourself too much when it comes to foods. You can still enjoy the dishes that you like but with control and moderation.

<u>Keep in mind:</u>

- Your health would definitely benefit from a good mix of nutrient-filled foods that are both alkaline and acid-forming. This would be the most ideal thing for anyone and the best thing is that it isn't hard to achieve at all.

Remember that you don't have to go over the top and completely switch up your diet. What you need to do, however, is get to the very core and make sure you have a solid foundation of good foods there.

Chapter 5: Acidic Foods And The Negative Effects They Have On Energy Levels

Generally, some of the most acidic foods out there won't seem that way to you at first glance. For example, there are a lot of fruits that are actually nutritious but when consumed in great amounts can actually turn pretty acidic. Good examples of these are bananas and melons. The same can be said for vegetables; there are acidic ones that you actually consume on a daily basis.

But how do these affect your energy levels?

Excessive amounts of acid in your body can begin to deplete oxygen supply, something that your cells need in order to function properly. If your cells are not working efficiently, you'll begin to notice changes in your energy level as well as immunity to even the most common illnesses.

A highly acidic environment also destroys healthy cells and impairs the body's ability to produce more; thus leading to a disruption in your bodily functions. This can affect your energy as well as your overall health.

Common symptoms of this includes:

- Unusual lethargy
- Inability to focus properly
- Easily depleted energy even with just minor activity

Highly acidic foods that you should stay away from or eat much less of include:

- Carbonated, high sugar content drinks
- Caffeinated drinks
- Chocolates
- Fatty foods

Another thing to remember is that over-acidity leads to the body leeching alkaline minerals from our bones, tissues and muscles in order to try and maintain the body's delicate pH balance. When this happens, it renders our body and cellular metabolism inefficient, thus making us feel tired and slugging.

It also inhibits the body's ability to use any stored up energy and reserves; but take note that that's just the beginning of the problem. In time, with the calcium being drained from our bones constantly, osteoporosis will set in.

Chapter 6: Alkaline Superfoods And How They Naturally Give Our Bodies More Energy

Here are some of the healthiest alkaline-forming superfoods that will provide us with better energy as well as boost our overall health:

Root vegetables – Radishes, turnips, carrots, rutabaga, horseradish and beets should become staples in your everyday diet. They are easy to prepare and are also richer in minerals when compared to other vegetables.

Cruciferous vegetables – Cabbages, broccoli, Brussels sprouts and cauliflower fall under this category. They are delicious and can be cooked in a number of different ways.

Leafy Green Veggies – These include kale, spinach, turnip greens and Swiss chard. All are, of course, considered favourites by many health and green eating buffs. They are rich in vitamin content and also contain a bunch of other good things such as: antioxidants, phytochemicals and fiber. Lastly, they also help in improving both vision and digestion.

Garlic – Considered by experts as a miracle food, garlic certainly brings a lot of good stuff to the table. Not only is it alkaline-forming, it also helps in improving both cardiovascular as well as immune health by lowering your blood pressure. It also detoxifies the liver as well as fights off any infection you might have in your body. An apple a day? How about a garlic a day definitely keeps the doctor away?

Cayenne Peppers – Do you like spicy dishes? If so, you'll be glad to know that you're on the right track when it comes to getting started with an alkaline diet. Tropical peppers contain certain enzymes that are actually essential to your endocrinal function. Besides this, it is alkaline-forming and also has antibacterial properties that would help fight off any internal infections that you might have. If you're typically stressed out over work, it is also a helpful agent when it comes to flushing out free radicals that often cause illnesses.

Lemon –This might just be the most alkalizing food of them all. It is also a natural disinfectant, capable of healing wounds and preventing infection. If you're experiencing hyperacidity, it would be able to provide you with immediate relief as it effectively counteracts the effects of acidity and neutralizes it in no time at all. Besides that, it can also help in relieving colds, coughs, flu and even heartburn.

Those are just a few of the alkaline-forming superfoods that you could easily add to any meal or have on hand as a snack. They're all healthy and easy to prepare. The best bit? There are numerous things that you can do with them too. So if you're keen on cooking, you'll be able to flex your creativity with these healthy ingredients.

Chapter 7: Alkaline/Acid Foods And How They Affect Fat Burning And Losing Weight

Alright, now that we all know how alkaline and acidic foods affect our overall health, let's talk about how it can help us effectively lose weight. You may not think much of it but eating highly acidic foods actually largely contribute to why we gain weight.

Here's a quick rundown of how it happens.

- If you become acidic, one way through which your body deals with it is by storing it in blood cells. This way, it becomes easier to flush out. However, too much acid can also bring about an excess amount of fat cells stores, hence making you gain weight.

- We've already pointed out the fact that acidity will make your cells unhealthy and if that happens, they become less efficient when performing their specific tasks. This also includes getting rid of fat from your body. In time, this will accumulate and you'll start seeing physical manifestations of the fat stores in your body.

- Exercising is one of the best ways to lose weight; however, acidity can completely zap your energy, thus leaving you unable to work out as much as you would like. In fact, because you start feeling more lethargic, physical work would only strain you much easier.

- Unhealthy cells also mean that they will not be able to properly absorb your body's much needed nutrients from the foods you eat. So even if you eat a lot, you won't end up feeling satisfied simply because your body feels as if it's not enough or that it isn't getting what it needs. Overeating and a lack of proper exercise can only lead to one thing: weight gain.

Some of the most acidic foods that can also cause weight gain include sweets, foods made with white flour, carbonated beverages, sodas, fast food meals, too much meat (especially red meat), coffee as well as most processed and canned foods.

So how do you counteract all of that? To do this, you will need to put your blood pH back into proper balance by adding more alkaline-forming foods into your diet. Alkaline foods bring great benefits to the table when it comes to weight loss and keeping the pounds off. Let me break things down for you:

- It is not unusual for people to experience digestion problems when they are acidic. However, if you can keep your blood pH at the right level, you'll be able to avoid that as well as flush out the toxins from your body more effectively.

- A properly alkaline body results to healthier cell production. **This is certainly beneficial when it comes to elevating your energy.** You wouldn't feel lethargic anymore and you will be able to exercise as much as you need during the day. Because oxygen is efficiently spread throughout your body, any harmful free radicals that might be sapping you of your energy will also be flushed out as you work out.

- Healthy cells also mean efficient nutrient absorption from the foods you eat. If your body is able to fully absorb what it needs from the foods you consume, then you'll feel satisfied and full quickly. This will help you avoid overeating. The good news is that if you stick to the good kinds of food products, then you can also easily avoid the unnecessary intake of fats.

- You'll be able to clean up your diet. No more fast foods or any fat-heavy foods that provide you with very little in terms of energy and nutrients and yet make you gain weight like crazy. Simply consuming less of refined carbs such as pasta and foods with flour can make a significant difference when it comes to your weight loss.

Chapter 8: Recommended Alkaline Foods For Weight Loss

Are you looking for more effective ways to eat well while also losing weight at the same time? Well, here are a few alkaline foods that you should add into your daily diet or meal plan:

- Almonds and almond milk
- amaranth
- artichokes
- arugula
- asparagus
- avocado and avocado oil
- beetroot
- broccoli
- Brussels sprouts
- buckwheat
- cabbage
- carrots
- cauliflower
- celery
- chia
- coconut
- collard greens
- cucumber
- eggplant
- endive
- flax seeds
- goat's milk
- green beans
- kale
- kelp
- lentils
- lettuce
- lima beans,
- mung beans
- mustard greens
- new potatoes
- olive oil

- pumpkin
- quinoa
- radish
- red beans
- rhubarb
- soybeans
- spinach
- sprouts
- squash
- sweet potato
- Swiss chard
- tofu
- tomatoes
- watercress
- wheat grass
- zucchini

When it comes to dieting, remember that you don't have to limit yourself to just these foods alone. However, they do serve as a great alkaline base for the rest of your diet. You need not completely remove your favourites from your life; but you need to find the right balance. Having this would allow you to not just lose weight but also keep it off.

A little indulgence every now and then is completely fine; but it would be even better if you can find an alkaline alternative for it. Trust us when we say that there are healthier substitutes to your favourite foods. Some of these substitutes are also as delicious as your favourites. It's all about getting creative when preparing your meals.

Chapter 9: Recommended Alkaline Foods For Beautiful Skin And A Youthful Appearance

Alkaline diet for better skin? Quite the unusual notion, right? As it turns out, this is not quite the case. In fact, it makes a lot of sense considering that what you consume on a daily basis would eventually affect your body from the inside to the outside. Once you detoxify your body from within, the changes would also manifest itself on your skin. Not only will you get better and healthier-looking skin, you can also delay aging.

Among the culprits for premature skin aging are free radicals. They are harmful toxins that can also cause different illnesses. We get these from our environment and unless you're planning on staying indoors for the rest of your life, your body will absorb them at some point. This isn't too bad as long as your body is capable of flushing them out but that's when problems arise. If you're acidic, your cells are less capable of getting rid of these free radicals so they continuously rise in number until you begin to see and feel the effects physically. Ask yourself:

- Have you been breaking out a lot lately?
- Do you have dry and flaky skin?
- Do you have brittle hair?
- Does your skin look pallid and lifeless?

If you answered yes to more than two of those questions, then don't fret! There are ways to turn things around and achieve clearer skin without the use of any creams or serums. All you need to do is change up your diet for the better. To help you with that, here are some of the recommended alkaline foods when it comes to getting clearer and healthier skin:

- Start by eating lots of fresh and green veggies with high water content. Try and have these veggies with your every meal. This should keep your skin nourished from the inside. Healthy salads or steamed veggies are a great start for this. Avocadoes and tomatoes are known to be excellent for the skin as well. As much as possible, however, do try to eat them raw.

- Alkaline water is good for your body and your skin. The best bit is that it's very easy to make them at home using ingredients that you prefer. Making sure that you're well hydrated throughout the day is one way to keep your skin nourished. Proper hydration also improves the ability of your body to flush out harmful toxins. However, adding some elements of alkalinity to water can make it even better. Quick fact: In some places like Seoul, they actually use unflavoured alkaline water to wash their faces. It is said that it moisturizes the skin efficiently and leaves it with a dewy glow.

- Green juices. These juices are great if you want to receive your daily recommended dosage of greens without taking up a whole lot of time for preparation. This is great if you're always in a hurry in the morning. A bit of kale and some spinach should put you on the right track. If you have some pH drops or other alkaline supplements available, then you can also go ahead and add them all in.

- Seaweed is also a great source of alkaline, not to mention it's also very good for the skin. In fact, it is often used in many skin creams because of its moisturizing effect. Of course, in this case, you can do it both ways. Have it with some of your meals and if you're keen, use one as a mask as well. Remember that our skin can absorb the nutrients from whatever we use on it so do make sure that you use an all-natural product for this purpose.

- Yogurt. Greek yogurt, in particular, is not only alkaline-forming but is also beneficial to your skin. Having it for breakfast with a few berries would certainly help boost your overall skin health. Blueberries are great for this purpose as they are known to have detoxifying qualities, something that you'll certainly benefit from as well.

- Green and yellow peppers. Have you been noticing crow's feet around your eyes? Well, you'll be glad to know that peppers can help with that. It can help decrease your sensitivity to UV rays as well as provide your skin with lots of antioxidants to help in fighting off free radicals. Two cups of green and yellow peppers every day is the recommended amount.

- Sunflower seeds are also great for this purpose. They are loaded with vitamin E and are capable of keeping your skin supple as well as protecting the top layers from the sun. Simply eat a handful daily and you'll be able to reap its benefits.

- Often relegated to being a breakfast food, oatmeal also has a number of skin benefits that you will surely enjoy. Steel cut oatmeal, in particular, is much less processed when compared to other varieties so if you're choosing one, then go for this variety. It contains more vitamins and takes longer to breakdown; hence it can keep your blood sugar level more stable. Keep in mind that an elevated blood sugar is not only bad for your health but for your skin as well-- it can contribute to the formation of wrinkles.

So there you have it, just a few examples of the top choices when it comes to alkaline-forming foods that are also great for your skin. Remember, always choose the natural and organic variety for this purpose since this can retain most of the nutrients that your body needs.

Chapter 10: Recommended Alkaline Foods For Increasing Energy, Health And Longevity

First off, let's talk about energy. If your diet is mostly comprised of fast food take-outs and meats, then it wouldn't be too surprising if you constantly experience bouts of lethargy. This is one of the most common symptoms brought on by a highly acidic diet. Not only that, it can also significantly affect your mood. Lethargy coupled with constant mood drops and irritability are sure signs that you need to switch up your diet. So, what should be at the top of your list when it comes to alkaline and energizing foods? Here's a short list:

Nuts and seeds – These are great sources of energizing protein as well as magnesium. Both nuts and seeds help in converting sugar from our foods to energy and increase the blood flow to our brain. Almonds and almond milk are also great for this purpose, especially if you're looking for a healthy, dairy substitute. Brazil nuts are great sources of selenium which does not only help with energy but also with improving your mood.

Fresh fruits -Some fruits are considered acidic so you need to be careful when it comes to choosing. One of the most alkalizing fruits is apple. Do you know that eating one a day actually helps in keeping the sleepiness away? Berries can also increase your energy levels throughout the day which makes them one of the best healthy snacks to carry around in place of an energy bar.

Leafy greens – The iron from these foods helps in transporting as well as storing oxygen in your body. In fact, without a proper amount of iron, we will be greatly lacking in energy. Organic leafy greens such as collard greens, broccoli, lettuce and spinach are all great sources of iron for your body. Have them raw in salads or add them to your smoothies, either way they will pack a punch when it comes to boosting your energy.

Now, let's talk about health. All over the world, more and more people are turning to greener and healthier ways of living as well as eating. These days, more people are conscious about what they consume and how these foods affect their body. We've already provided you with a list of the right foods to eat so this time, let's talk about those that you should avoid or have less of in order to maintain your good health and boost your longevity.

- Avoid processed grains as well as sugar as much as you can. These two are the most common culprits when it comes to making your body acidic. Try and limit them as much as you can or switch to healthier alternatives such as quinoa, wild rice and millet.

- East less dairy and meat. These are also quite acidifying especially if you have them in huge amounts and on a daily basis. The cheeseburgers you have for lunch and even dinner? They will eventually make you sick. Look for healthier protein food alternatives such as goat milk and goat cheese, almonds and soy products.

- Avoid all artificial sweeteners. There are many alternatives to these. Stevia is the most commonly used but you can also try pure maple sugar or raw sugar as other options. You may not notice it but you consume a significant amount of artificial sweeteners on a daily basis; in your coffee, to sweeten your juices and smoothies -- all of these things will eventually take their toll on your body so do switch to something healthier.

- Tone down your caffeine intake. If you need coffee to perk you up every morning and then a few more cups to keep you going throughout the day, then you may be hastening acidosis in your body. If you're after an energy boost, there are a number of green smoothies that you can have in place of this.

- Balance. Last but certainly not the least, you need to find a proper balance in your diet. Keep in mind that too much alkalinity can actually be bad for your body. While you're supposed to avoid certain foods, it doesn't mean that you have to completely eliminate them from your diet. Just make sure that you consume the more acidic foods in moderation. Remember, your diet should be 80% alkaline and 20% acidic.

Cancer Prevention:

When talking about longevity, it is important to remember that prevention will always be better than finding a cure for what ails you. A major benefit of keeping your body pH properly balanced is that it actually aids in lowering your cancer risks. If your body remains highly acidic all the time, then your oxygen levels are significantly lower and cellular metabolism eventually stops.

This can then lead to the development of cancer cells. Maintaining alkalinity will encourage healthier cell turnover and this is the key to preventing cancer and keeping yourself healthy for the long term.

Conclusion

Thank you again for purchasing this book on getting started with alkaline foods and learning more about the health benefits!

I am extremely excited to pass this information along to you, and I am so happy that you now have read and can hopefully implement these strategies going forward.

I hope this book was able to help you understand what alkaline foods are and how you can apply them to your body and increase your health. The next step is to get started using this information and to hopefully live a better, healthier and longer life.

Please don't be someone who just reads this information and doesn't apply it, the strategies in this book will only benefit you if you use them! If you know of anyone else that could benefit from the information presented here please inform them of this book.

Finally, if you enjoyed this book and feel it has added value to your life in any way, please take the time to share your thoughts and post a review on Amazon. It'd be greatly appreciated!

Thank you and good luck!

Preview Of:

Ultimate Coconut Oil Guide!

Coconut Oil

Coconut Oil Recipes For Organic Skin Care And Natural Beauty, Clean Eating For Weight Loss, Shinning Hair, Better Brain Function And Overall Health!

Introduction

I want to thank you and congratulate you for purchasing the book, *Coconut Oil: Ultimate Coconut Oil Guide! - Coconut Oil Recipes For Organic Skin Care And Natural Beauty, Clean Eating For Weight Loss, Shining Hair, Better Brain Function And Overall Health!*

This book contains proven steps and strategies on how you can take full advantage of the beauty, weight loss and health benefits that coconut oil has to offer. Through this book, you will learn more about:

- What makes coconut oil healthy?
- How it can help you get better, more glowing skin.
- Its effects on your hair and making healthier.
- Can coconut oil improve your brain function?
- Weight loss benefits and how it can boost your metabolism.
- Coconut oil and how it can help treat different illnesses.
- Recipes for both your diet as well as organic skin care.
- How to choose the right coconut oil for your needs.

We hope that through this book, you'll be able to recognize the amount of potential that a single bottle of coconut oil contains.

Thanks again for purchasing this book, I hope you enjoy it!

Chapter 1: Coconut Oil For Natural Beauty And Health

These days, more and more people are becoming aware of the effects that chemically manufactured products has on their bodies. As such, many of them have turned to a greener, more organic lifestyle that advocates going all natural when it comes to their food as well as the different products that they use on their bodies.

This isn't surprising, of course, considering the fact that there are a number of illnesses which are associated with constant use of synthetic and often chemical-laden skin and health products. There are certain risks that one must bear when using it; risks which can be avoided altogether if one were to switch over to something that's a bit closer to nature.

The coconut oil is a favourite among health buffs as it is one of those by-products that can be used in a multitude of ways. On one hand, it can be eaten and taken as a supplement which would boost your overall health. On the other, it can be applied topically and used as a beauty product as well as a means of treating certain skin issues.

You get all of these benefits but without worrying about its harmful effects to the body.

Why is it considered one of the best natural remedies out there?

It's all in the composition. About 99% of it is composed of saturated fats (which, in this case isn't as bad as it sounds) as well as traces of polyunsaturated fatty acids and monosaturated fatty acids. Virgin coconut oil retains a higher amount of the good stuff thus it is also valued higher.

It also contains lauric acid and quite a generous amount of it at that. When digested by the body, this would turn into monolaurin and is very beneficial when it comes to dealing with different bacteria and viruses. Diseases such as influenza and herpes are just two of the things that coconut oil can cure in a jiff. A tablespoon of it a day keeps the doctor away, so to speak.

Besides these, it is also one of the most powerful inhibitors of quite a number of different pathogenic organisms ranging from your usual viruses to even protozoa. All of this, of course, is attributed to its high lauric acid content.

For beauty and skincare

Coconut can also be used for cosmetic or skin care purposes. We'll get to the specifics of this in later chapters but to quickly summarize, it is often used for: Hair care, skin care, nails, lips as well as treating different skin issues such as psoriasis. It helps keep the skin youthful and glowing as well as protect it from harmful UV rays.

Thanks for Previewing My Exciting Book Entitled:

"Coconut Oil: Ultimate Coconut Oil Guide! Coconut Oil Recipes For Organic Skin Care And Natural Beauty, Clean Eating For Weight Loss, Shinning Hair, Better Brain Function And Overall Health!"

To purchase this book, simply go to the Amazon Kindle store and simply search:

"COCONUT OIL"

Then just scroll down until you see my book. You will know it is mine because you will see my name "Sarah Brooks" underneath the title.

Alternatively, you can visit my author page on Amazon to see this book and other work I have done. Thanks so much, and please don't forget your free bonuses

DON'T LEAVE YET! - CHECK OUT YOUR FREE BONUSES BELOW!

Free Bonus Offer: Get Free Access To The LiveFitVIP.com VIP Newsletter!

Once you enter your email address you will immediately get free access to this awesome newsletter! But wait, right now if you join now for free you will also get free access to the "The 7 Keys To Body Transformation" free EBook!

To claim both your FREE VIP NEWSLETTER MEMBERSHIP and your FREE BONUS EBook on THE 7 KEYS TO BODY TRANSFORMATION!

Just Go To:

www.liveFitVIP.com